Alexander Kruglov, Alexander Vasilyev,
Veronica Sherman

Human Dynamic Homeostasis Control Matrix in the Norm with Psychophysiological Aspects

International Medical Research and Development Corporation
New York
2016

Alexander Kruglov, Alexander Vasilyev, Veronica Sherman

HUMAN DYNAMIC HOMEOSTASIS CONTROL MATRIX IN THE NORM WITH PSYCHOPHYSIOLOGICAL ASPECTS

First paperback edition printed in 2016.

Published by International Medical Research and Development Corporation.
www.imrdcorp.org

Edited by Marietta Eliseyeva, PhD, ScD
Production Manager: Paul Edelstein

Library of Congress Control Number: 2016930813
ISBN: 978-0-692-61998-8
10 9 8 7 6 5 4 3 2 1

Printed in the United States of America
2016

To Professor George Gebel, Friend and Teacher,
dedicated with admiration and gratitude

Alexander Kruglov, Alexander Vasilyev, Veronica Sherman

HUMAN DYNAMIC HOMEOSTASIS CONTROL MATRIX IN THE NORM WITH PSYCHOPHYSIOLOGICAL ASPECTS

International Medical Research and Development Corporation
www.imrdcorp.org

About the Authors

Alexander Kruglov

Doctor of medical sciences. Expert in the field of physiology, pathophysiology, psychophysiology, and psychiatry. Author of over 220 publications, including 2 monographs. Deputy Director of Central Research Institute of Radiation Diagnosis. Moscow, the Russian Federation.

Alexander Vasilyev

Professor of medicine, Academician of the Russian Academy of Sciences. Author of over 320 publications including 16 monographs. Head of Department of the Radiology of the Moscow State University of Medicine and Dentistry.

Veronica Sherman

Veronica Sherman earned her bachelor's degree in biology and pharmacology at Nova Southern Eastern University. She is a pharmacologist in critical care at Memorial Hospital News (Florida) and an expert in practical implementation of theoretical models in biology.

CONTENTS

ABBREVIATION

Ao - aorta
BP - blood pressure
CI - confidence interval ratio
CVBF- cerebral venous blood flow
CASs - carotid artery siphons
CO - cardiac minute output
DP - diastolic pressure
Er – erythrocyte
F.d.p. - final diastolic pressure of the right ventricle
F-n – fibrinogen
GDB - goal-directed behavior
ICP - intracranial pressure
IVP - intracranial venous blood pressure
IJV - internal jugular vein
LV - left ventricle
M - mean value
MP - medium pressure
Max - maximum value
Min - minimum value
MG - motivational gradient
N – Norm
O_2-$AVDO_2$ - arterio-venous oxygen content difference
P-n – protein
Pl – plasma
PP - pulse pressure
RA - right atrium
RV - right ventricle
SS - sigmoid sinus
SinP - sigmoid sinus pressure
SVC - superior vena cava
SP - systolic pressure
SV - stroke volume
SAH - sustained arterial hypertension
ST - subjective time

CHAPTER 1.

DYNAMIC HOMEOSTASIS CONTROL MATRIX IN HEALTHY HUMANS AS COMPARED TO ARTERIAL HYPERTENSION

The research has been undertaken to study the relationship between the biochemical and hemodynamic parameters of the bloodstream, their impact on the cerebral venous blood flow (CVBF), on the interaction between hemodynamics of CVBF and the blood flow in the right atrium (RA), right ventricle (RV), left ventricle (LV), and the aortic chamber in apparently healthy people (the norm) as compared with patients suffering from sustained arterial hypertension (SAH).

The catheterization through the probe secured at the level of the superior bulb of the internal jugular vein (IJV) made it possible to obtain hemodynamic and biochemical values of CVBF without admixture of extracranial blood. Arterial blood was taken from the thoracic aorta. The correlation and factor analyses were conducted to study the relationship between the biochemical characteristics of the blood flow and the hemodynamic values of the cerebral blood inflow and outflow in apparently healthy people and to compare them with the respective characteristics of the SAH group. The obtained results suggested the existence of the primary homeostatic control of the factors determining rheological and thrombogenic properties of blood (involved in development of ischemic cardiac and cerebral events); regulation of brain gas exchange and intracranial venous pressure by the minimum level of pressure in the cerebral outflow pathway—the pressure in RA; and the existence of synergistic relationships between the studied biochemical and hemodynamic characteristics that form the human homeostasis control matrix in the norm. The comparison of the matrix parameters with the respective parameters in SAH revealed a drastic change in the entire set of relationships typical of the norm, including loss of control of viscosity characteristics, cerebral regulation by the minimum pressure in the cerebral outflow pathway, and change in the entire range of endogenous relationships of the homeostatic control. The choice of the research area is explained by the lack of conceptual uniformity of the present-day ideas of the relationship between hemodynamics and the biochemistry of intracranial and intracerebral blood flow, and characteristics of the blood inflowing and outflowing from the brain.

The **objective** of the research was to identify a relationship between biochemical characteristics of blood inflowing and outflowing from the brain, and their correlation with the hemodynamics of the studied organs in healthy people, to prove the relationship between the qualitative changes in the biochemical blood composition and certain risk factors contributing to the development of brain ischemic conditions as well as to the development of coagulation complications associated with CVBF observed in SAH. For our research purposes, we opted for the hemodynamic pathway: LV — Ao (aorta) — CVBF — SS (sigmoid sinus) — RA — RV: in other words, the pathway locating the arterial venous difference (AVD) of cerebral O_2 oxygen content difference, which is seen as the main indicator of the CVBF adequacy and cerebral metabolism.

Methods

All of the research through which we received the results discussed in this chapter, was conducted in the same laboratory and with the help of the same methods. The data obtained by using the catheterization performed with a probe secured at the level of the superior bulb of IJV show blood pressure levels in the cerebral venous system, in SS. The collected blood samples without admixture of the extracranial blood are biochemically indicative of the cerebral metabolism. We performed the catheterization of LV, Ao, IJV, SVC (superior vena cava), RA, and RV; during the procedure the pressure levels were recorded and blood samples were collected. The catheterization was performed by percutaneous puncture of the right femoral artery and the right femoral vein under local anesthesia, using the Seldinger technique. A vein dilator was used during the vein puncture. The catheter reached the aforesaid parts of the cardiovascular system. The blood pressure values were recorded for the thoracic aorta. The studies were monitored by using radiography equipment.

The results for assessment were obtained from the studies conducted on apparently healthy people who were thoroughly examined in hospital before complex reconstructive maxillofacial surgery (the data were given in our earlier studies). The total number of the examined people was 60 (48 men and 12 women). The age of 52 of those people ranged from 20 to 45 (the average age was 28.8), and 8 people were over 45 years old.

The reference group consisted of patients suffering from SAH degree 2. All examined patients had long-term SAH resistant to therapy. The preliminary test did not reveal any significant differences in qualitative characteristics of the hemodynamic and biochemical blood parameters in the patients; we can consider the examined group as homogeneous and having SAH. The total number of patients was 61(43 men and 18 women). Two patients were under 20 years old; the age of 39 patients ranged from 20 to 45; 11 patients were 45 to 60 years old; 9 patients were over 60. The average age was 43.8 years; the average duration of the disease was 11.5 years. All the patients had medical pre-treatment. As there was no effect from the pre-treatment, the patients were hospitalized to be further examined for surgical treatment options. All the patients were examined when they had SAH.

The linear and factor statistical analysis was performed with consideration for significant correlation coefficients ($P<0.05$). All blood pressure values are given in mmHg.

Results and Discussion

When assessing the results, we took into consideration some principles of the regulation theory: If there is a multitude of functional stability parameters, the self-regulating homeostatic system will find this multitude and restore the stability of the system, regardless of any changes in the environment. The range of physiological changes, within which the life activity that is optimum for the new environment can be performed, is seen as normal.

Therefore, for the person whose body functions in the changed environment (long-lasting arterial hypertension), finding the blood pressure levels at the exit from the intracranial venous system draining blood from the brain within the "normal range" corresponds to a stable pattern of functioning.

To define boundaries of the normal range we used the confidence interval boundaries set for each parameter and value; these boundaries define the range within which the probability of the relevant parameter value is 95%. Changes in the confidence interval boundaries were seen as indicators of changing stability of the system and, consequently, of its adaptive properties (Tables 1-5).

Table 1.
The pressure levels in the sigmoid sinus

		SP	DP	PP	MP
N	M	10.5	8.3	2.4	9.4
	CI	2.2	1.8	0.75	2.2
	Max	21.6	16.8	4.2	18.9
	Min	6	3.9	0.5	4.9
SAH		SP	DP	PP	MP
	M	11.5	7.7	3.8	10,1
	m	3.2	2.9	1.4	3.9
	Max	22.6	19.2	7	20.4
	Min	3.9	2.1	1.3	2.4

Table 2.
Pressure levels in the internal jugular vein

		SP	DP	PP	MP
N	M	7.3	5.5	2.1	6.7
	CI	1.1	1	0.6	1.3
	Max	13.8	10.5	5.1	11.7
	Min	2.4	2	0.2	1.4
SAH		SP	DP	PP	MP
	M	8.7	6.3	2.6	7.2
	CI	3.4	3,3	1.1	3.2
	Max	21	14.6	6.4	15.7
	Min	2.4	0.5	1.2	2.1

The above data show that the maximum, minimum and mean pressure levels of SAH patients are within the normal range typical of the norm in the intra- and extracranial venous systems transporting the blood outflow from the brain. In SAH patients, IVP reaches the level where the vein, seen in cross-sectional view, changes its shape from elliptical into cylindrical (the maximum blood flow). Note that there is a constant pressure differential between the intra- and extracranial venous systems, though the IJV pressure levels are prone to change (affected by the intrathoracic and barometric pressure), thus being indicative of the SinP development, taking into account the IJV pressure and its underlying factors.

Table 3.

Pressure levels in the aorta

		SP	DP	PP	MP
N	M	114	71	40.3	92.6
	CI	4.5	3.8	3.5	5.1
	Max	147	87	65	115
	Min	90	50	21	70
SAH		SP	DP	PP	MP
	M	180	101	79	137
	CI	31	21	22	23
	Max	270	155	144	210
	Min	150	78	40	96

Although the above data are well-known and can be found in many studies, we need them for more detailed description of the obtained results.

For many years, various authors [1-7] have been referring to electrolytes, gases and acid-base parameters when talking about active CBF regulators. We have examined the values of the following parameters: content levels of plasma electrolytes (Pl) and red blood cells (Er), blood gases (pO_2, pCO_2), acid-base composition (ABC - pH, SB), blood proteins: hemoglobin (Hb), fibrinogen (F-n), total protein (P-n), arterial venous difference ($AVDO_2$), and hematocrit (Ht).

Table 4.

Biochemical values of the cerebral blood outflow (SS)

		K pl	K er	Na pl	Na er	pH	pCO_2	SB	pO_2	HBO_2	HB	Ht	F-n	P-n	$AVDO_2$
N	M	3.9	80.6	136.2	31.1	7.32	46	21.9	50.7	73	13.1	46	292	7.7	4.2
	CI	0.2	1.9	3.1	2.5	0.02	2	0.9	7.7	4.8	0.9	3.7	41	0.5	0.5
	Max	5.1	86.3	146.5	37.5	7.44	62	27.5	64	85	15.8	54	488	8.9	7.2
	Min	3.1	70.8	117	20	7.14	22	15.5	30	51	9.8	32	177	6.6	1.4
SAH		K pl	K er	Na pl	Na er	pH	pCO_2	SB	pO_2	HBO_2	HB	Ht	F-n	P-n	$AVDO_2$
	M	4.3	78.3	132.2	28.7	7.31	45.4	23.4	52	68	12.4	45	329	7.6	4.3
	CI	1.4	4.4	5.8	2.6	0.06	7.4	7.3	9.7	6.6	1.4	3.6	47	0.5	1.4
	Max	9.6	95.2	150	40.5	7.47	61	33	68	83	16.2	59	444	8.9	9.6
	Min	1.7	70.9	118.5	22.3	7.09	34	15	35	55	10.2	37	222	6.5	1.7

As for electrolytes, the SAH group showed expansion of the confidence interval boundaries as compared to norm. The results are consistent with the data of the well-known studies that point out the correlation between electrolytes in norm and SAH. The changes in gases (O_2, CO_2) representing the qualitative characteristics of the cerebral metabolism are also insignificant and do not reach limit values, which can cause physiological responses of the CBF vascular system. Hb, Ht, F-n, and P-n are the same in both groups. When the balance of mean, maximum, and minimum values is retained, for ABC parameters the SAH group demonstrates significant changes in the boundaries of the confidence interval. The mean $AVDO_2$ values show no difference, thus evidencing that CBF is adequate to cerebral metabolism when the confidence interval boundaries expand significantly.

We can conclude that the changes in the examined biochemical characteristics of the cerebral blood outflow, which were measured against the mean values, are not significant and are within the normal range in SAH patients. On the other hand, we should point out an increase in the confidence interval as compared to the norm parameters.

Table 5.

Biochemical parameters of the cerebral blood inflow (Ao)

		K pl	K er	Na pl	Na er	pH	pCO_2	SB	pO_2	HBO_2	HB	Ht	F-n	P-n
N	M	3.9	80.5	135	31.4	7.37	39	22	95	94	13.1	45.8	294	7.5
	CI	0.2	2.3	3.5	1.9	0.02	2.4	1	1.4	1.1	1.1	2.1	45	0.5
	Max	4.6	91.3	160	38.8	7.46	55	28.5	102	100	22	55	444	8.9
	Min	2.9	66.3	122	23.8	7.21	25	15	84	83	9.5	36	132	5.9
SAH		K pl	K er	Na pl	Na er	pH	pCO_2	SB	pO_2	HBO_2	HB	Ht	F-n	P-n
	M	3.8	77.8	134.4	30.2	7.36	39	22	93	94	12.5	43	321	7.65
	CI	0.6	4.6	5.7	3.3	0.06	8.7	3.2	6.9	2.4	1.4	2.2	49	0.5
	Max	5.3	91.3	147.5	39.3	7.5	67	31	100	98	16.2	50	444	8.3
	Min	2.5	70	124	24.4	7.22	25	12.5	85	88	10	37	200	6.6

For electrolytes, pH, SB and blood gases (pO_2, pCO_2), expansion of the confidence interval boundaries is noted. HbO_2, Hb, Ht, F-n, and P-n of both groups do not show any significant differences.

We can summarize the cerebral blood inflow and outflow data as follows: the changes in the content levels of biochemical substances, which were measured against the mean values, are insignificant both in the norm and SAH, remaining within the normal range. The conformity between the quantitative biochemical cerebral blood inflow and outflow characteristics in the reference and SAH group implies that the relationships between these substances can be changed in the blood flow.

The results of the correlation analysis, which are given in the tables, suggest an interrelationship between the studied characteristics and values, their changes, and their tendencies (Table 6-7).

Table 6.

Analysis of the biochemical relationship for cerebral blood outflow (SS)

		K pl	K er	Na pl	Na er	pH	pCO_2	SB	pO_2	HBO_2	HB	Ht	F-n	P-n
N	K er			/+/	/+/	/-/			/+/					
	Ht			/+/		/+/								
	F-n	/+/						/+/						/-/
	P-n			/+/						/-/		/+/	/-/	
	Hb				/-/									
SAH		K pl	K er	Na pl	Na er	pH	pCO_2	SB	pO_2	HBO_2	HB	Ht	F-n	P-n
	K er									/+/				
	Ht						/+/				/+/			
	F-n								/-/		/-/			
	P-n			/-/									/+/	
	Hb											/+/	/-/	

Table 7.

Analysis of the biochemical relationship for cerebral blood inflow

		K pl	K er	Na pl	Na er	pH	pCO_2	SB	pO_2	HBO_2	HB	Ht	F-n	P-n
N	K er			/-/	/+/				/+/					
	Ht			/-/							/+/		/+/	
	F-n			/-/		/+/			/-/		/+/	/+/		/+/
	P-n			/+/		/-/			/+/	/-/	/-/	/+/	/+/	
	Hb	/-/				/+/						/+/	/+/	/-/
SAH		K pl	K er	Na pl	Na er	pH	pCO_2	SB	pO_2	HBO_2	HB	Ht	F-n	P-n
	K er			/-/					/-/	/-/			/+/	
	Ht					/-/		/-/						/+/
	F-n		/+/	/-/										
	P-n				/-/				/-/			/+/		
	Hb			/+/		/-/		/-/		/-/				

The key distinction of the above data is their set of relationships—a group of structural parameters (Ker, Hb, Ht, P-n, F-n), which we refer to as the "basic complex of biochemical regulation" (BCBR) and which do not change during one cardio-cycle.

In our opinion, the following differences should be pointed out:

– in the cerebral blood inflow

Ker– the relationship with Naer is not revealed, which may be indicative of changes in the ATP activity and changes in the direction of energy metabolism through membranes. The pO_2 relationship is inverted; the inversion may be caused by changes in the erythrocyte membrane function. The relationship with F-n is formed. Ht retains the relationship with P-n. F-n retains the relationship with Na pl, while losing all other primary relationships, which may imply qualitative changes in F-n of SAH patients. P-n retains its relationship with Ht.

– in the cerebral blood outflow

Ker– the entire set of relationships has changed, except for a positive relationship with HbO_2, which shows the relationship between the oxygen-carrying function of red blood cells and the function of membranes. Hb demonstrates a negative relationship with F-n. Ht loses the entire primary set of relationships. F-n demonstrates both loss and changes in the entire set of primary relationships. P-n is characterized by the loss of the primary set and inverted relationships with F-n and Na pl.

As we believe that it is important to identify existing or absent correlation relationships of hemodynamics and biochemistry characteristics, we offer the data of the comparative analysis (Table 8).

Table 8.

The relationship between the SinP levels and biochemical parameters of cerebral blood inflow

		K pl	K er	Na pl	Na er	pH	pCO_2	SB	pO_2	HBO_2	HB	Ht	F-n	P-n
N	SP	/+/	/-/	/+/	/-/	/-/		/-/	/+/		/-/	/-/	/-/	/+/
	DP		/-/	/+/		/-/		/-/	/+/		/-/	/-/	/-/	/+/
	PP													
	MP		/-/			/-/		/-/	/+/		/-/	/-/	/-/	/+/
SAH		K pl	K er	Na pl	Na er	pH	pCO_2	SB	pO_2	HBO_2	HB	Ht	F-n	P-n
	SP					/-/			/-/	/+/	/+/			
	DP								/-/	/+/	/+/	/-/		
	PP		/-/	/-/			/+/	/-/						
	MP			/+/		/-/		/-/	/-/	/+/				

SAH is characterized by the following: a) inversion of the relationship with pO_2 for all pressure levels; b) inversion of the relationship with Hb; and c) new (positive) relationships with HbO_2 are formed for all pressure levels. The other BCBR relationships (K er, Hb, Ht, F-n, P-n) are absent in the SAH group. The SAH group is characterized by inversion of the relationships between the substances performing plasma (the most mobile) transportation of O_2 and by new relationships with the substances performing transportation of O_2 by formed elements of blood.

Thus, the levels of SinP in healthy people are positively interrelated with the factors affected by pressure—oncotic (P-n), gas (pO_2)—substances that have physical characteristics, i.e. the hydrodynamic pressure at the exit from the CVBF system, in SS changes in accordance with changes in the oncotic and gas pressure. In SAH patients, the interrelation between SinP and P-n (the evolutionary older type of pressure in multicellular biosystems) is absent; the relationship with pO_2 is inverted.

In contrast to P-n in the norm, relationships with cellular (Hb) and primarily with extracellular specialized protein (F-n) are negative (Table 9). The negative correlation with F-n, a major determinant of plasma viscosity, the substrate of clot formation, is indicative of increased outflow from venous collectors of the brain when the plasma viscosity is increased. When there is a fixed obstacle along the blood outflow path and the plasma viscosity is changed, SinP can serve as a regulator of the CBF adequacy. In SAH patients, the correlation between SinP and F-n is absent and the Hb relationship is inverted. It can be generally seen as loss of "cooperation" in protein-based regulation or reduction of the adaptation range.

Table 9.

The relationship between SinP levels and biochemical parameters of cerebral blood outflow

		K pl	K er	Na pl	Na er	pH	pCO_2	SB	pO_2	HBO_2	HB	Ht	F-n	P-n
N	SP	/-/		/+/		/-/		/-/			/-/		/-/	/+/
	DP	/-/		/+/		/-/	/+/	/-/			/-/		/-/	
	PP													
	MP	/-/		/+/		/-/		/-/			/-/		/-/	/+/
SAH		K pl	K er	Na pl	Na er	pH	pCO_2	SB	pO_2	HBO_2	HB	Ht	F-n	P-n
	SP		/+/		/-/		/+/			/+/	/+/			
	DP		/+/						/-/	/+/		/+/		
	PP				/-/	/-/			/+/			/-/		
	MP					/-/			/-/			/+/		

In healthy people, the complex of viscous dissipation (Hb, F-n) correlates with pressure levels in SS (Table 9).

Negative correlations prove that when the blood viscosity increases (risk of microcirculation impairment), SinP decreases, thus improving the outflow from the CBF zone. Absent in SAH patients is the correlation between SinP and the viscous dissipation parameters characterizing rheological properties of blood. In healthy people, the set of correlation relationships with BCBR is uniform for all SinP levels. Additional specific relationships are defined for each pressure level.

Patients suffering from SAH hardly have any relationships typical of the basic complex of biochemical regulation, demonstrating other and different relationships (Table 10).

Table 10.

The relationship between the pressure levels in IJV and the biochemical parameters of cerebral blood outflow

		K pl	K er	Na pl	Na er	pH	pCO_2	SB	pO_2	HBO_2	HB	Ht	F-n	P-n
N	SP					/-/	/+/		/-/			/+/	/+/	/-/
	DP	/-/		/+/			/-/		/-/				/-/	
	PP					/-/	/+/	/-/	/+/		/-/		/+/	
	MP	/-/	/+/	/-/				/-/					/-/	
SAH		K pl	K er	Na pl	Na er	pH	pCO_2	SB	pO_2	HBO_2	HB	Ht	F-n	P-n
	SP				/-/					/+/	/+/			/+/
	DP				/-/					/+/	/+/			/+/
	PP	/+/	/+/	/+/		/-/		/-/					/-/	
	MP				/-/					/+/	/+/			/+/

We can definitely speak about the completely changed composition and quality of correlation relationships of the extracranial venous bed in SAH patients. The relationship between all IJV pressure levels and the substances that characterize general and plasma viscosity in cerebral blood outflow (Ht, F-n) and rheological properties of blood disappears or becomes inverted. There is no longer a relationship with the end products of cerebral gas metabolism, which determine plasma tension of gases (pO_2, pCO_2); in other words, the entire complex of relationships with substances characterizing the physical and chemical composition of the cerebral blood outflow is changed. The aforesaid complex of biochemical substances is a permanent participant in adaptive mechanisms of the human body in acute and chronic stress conditions.

Thus, at all pressure levels at the entry and exit from the CBF system, the complex of correlation relationships with biochemical substances in the blood of SAH patients is fundamentally different from the complex of relationships typical of apparently healthy people. Changes in relationships of the biochemical composition of the blood flow are accompanied by similar endpoint events (SinP, $AVDO_2$ and other parameters) and imply that the balance is achieved in SAH patients through other methods. In other words, the aforesaid pressure levels and parameters are maintained within the normal range, while the biochemical status is qualitatively changed, along with the qualitatively changed methods of achieving stable SinP and $AVDO_2$ in SAH patients, as compared to norm.

Taking into consideration the specifics of the correlation analysis as a statistical method, we used it primarily as a tool for building pattern characteristics of the analyzed material, with due regard for modern-day concepts addressing relationships between intra- and extracranial hemodynamics and biochemistry. Based on the submitted data, we can state that in healthy people the hydrodynamic pressure in SS changes in accordance with changes in the oncotic pressure, gas pressure and blood viscosity parameters. In SAH patients, the above relationships are absent. We can assume that in SAH patients the commonly known increased stiffness of the walls of arterial vessels, including carotid artery siphons, as well as the above-mentioned changes in biochemical properties of blood cause changes in turbulent characteristics of the blood flow in intracerebral vessels. These changes result in changes in thermodynamic properties of the flow and cause changes in pulse pressure dissipation through the intracranial and intracerebral vascular bed. In other words, the relationship between the blood flow and cerebral tissue changes in the parameters characterizing physical properties of the interacting media: density, viscosity, capability of energy utilization, deformation, etc. Here we point out morphofunctional characteristics of the venous section of the cerebral vascular bed, as density (viscosity) is very significant for them: considerable size and tortuosity of pial veins, lacuna development when veins run into venous sinuses, trabecules, intersections, spikes in the lumen of venous sinuses, carotid artery siphons in the lumen of the cavernous sinus and veins running into it from sense organs; extensive receptor system. Changes in the rheological properties of blood in SAH patients, increased volumetric blood flow in the intracranial venous bed, increasing quantity of critical disturbances of a metabolic and hemodynamic nature result in impaired balance of blood as a metastable fluid and in dramatically increased risk of local transition from the liquid physical form into a polymerized form [8], i.e. risk of clot formation.

The obtained results suggested the conclusion that blood viscosity within the normal range can be seen as an initially regulated homeostasis parameter. In SAH, there is no homeostatic control of the factors determining the rheological and thrombogenic properties of blood as well as participating in development of ischemic cerebral events.

Note the increase in all RA pressure values in SAH patients as compared to healthy people with reference to mean values (P<0.01) outside the normal range (Table 11).

Table 11.
Pressure levels in RA and RV

Group		RA					RV	
		A	X	V	Y	M	FDP	Med.P
N	M	5.7	2.4	4.6	3.4	4.1	5.1	14.4
	CI	0.9	0.7	0.8	0.2	1.1	1.2	1.8
	Max	8.8	5.3	6.5	6.0	8.4	10	19.8
	Min	3.0	0	1,6	0	1.2	0	8,8
SAH	M	7.4	4.0	6.4	4.7	6.1	3.4	13.9
	CI	2.7	2.1	2.8	2.0	2.9	2.6	4.4
	Max	11.8	9.0	14.1	9.0	14.6	8.4	28
	Min	1.8	0	1.8	0	1.6	0	6.6

Note that in the norm the active process of LV (which was assessed by the Ao and LV systolic blood pressure (Table 12) and by the Ao pulse pressure) does not correlate with the SinP pulse pressure, thus demonstrating absence of any relationships.

Table 12.
Pressure levels in the aorta and left ventricle (LV)

Group		CO	SV	Ao				LV	
				SP	DP	PP	MP	SP	PP
N	M	10.9	128.4	114	71	40,3	92.6	108	100.5
	CI	1.3	22.4	4.5	3.8	3.5	5.1	6.4	7.1
	Max	18.7	186	147	87	65	115	130	130
	Min	5.5	80	90	50	21	70	90	85
SAH	M	11.1	147	180	101	79	137	180	168
	CI	3.1	38,9	31	21	22	23	34	28
	Max	21.7	246	270	155	144	210	260	248
	Min	5.3	50	150	78	40	96	150	138

The LV systolic pressure correlates negatively with the SS systolic, diastolic and mean blood pressure (Table 13).

Table 13.

Relationships between the SinP levels and the pressure levels in LV chamber

Group		Ao				CO	SV	SP LV	PP LV
		SP	DP	PP	MP				
N	SP				/+/	/-/		/-/	/-/
	DP		/+/		/+/	/-/		/-/	/-/
	PP		/-/						
	MP				/+/	/-/	/-/	/-/	/-/
SAH	SP			/+/					
	DP								
	PP	/+/	/+/	/+/	/+/		/-/	/+/	
	MP	/-/	/-/		/-/				

Therefore, in the norm, SinP development does not depend on the Ao pulse pressure, while being interrelated with the pressure levels in the arterial section of the vascular bed. In SAH patients, the relationship between SinP and the pressure in the left ventricle's aortic chamber is absent, while the LV active phase is interrelated with the SS pulse pressure (with the process responsible for the SinP differential). Thus, in the norm the SinP levels correlate with the phase of LV emptying: ejecting blood from LV into Ao; reaching the pressure maximum in the LV-Ao system, when the aortic valves are open; creating the pressure maximum for the head as a whole; and creating the wave process in Ao, when the nearest application point is the system of extra- and intracranial vessels (Table 14).

Table 14.

Relationships between the SinP and the central venous pressure levels

Group		RA					RV	
		Med.P	A	X	V	Y	FDP	Med.P
N	SP	/+/	/-/	/+/				/+/
	DP	/+/		/+/				/+/
	PP			/-/			/+/	
	MP	/+/		/+/		/+/	/-/	/+/
SAH	SP		/+/			/+/		
	DP		/+/			/+/		
	PP					/+/		
	MP					/+/	/+/	/+/

Note that in SAH patients, the complex of relationships is almost completely changed as compared to norm, and positive correlation relationships are formed with the Y-wave of RA for all SinP levels.

When the complex of correlation relationships changes significantly, SAH patients, in contrast to healthy people, start developing relationships with the X-collapse of RA, and these relationships are uniform for all IJV pressure levels (Table 15).

Table 15.
Relationships between the IJV pressure and the central venous pressure

Group		RA					RV	
		Med.P	A	X	V	Y	FDP	Med.P
N	SP	/+/	/-/		/-/	/+/		
	DP				/-/		/-/	/+/
	PP		/-/		/-/	/-/		/+/
	MP						/-/	
SAH	SP		/+/	/+/		/+/		/+/
	DP		/+/	/+/		/+/		
	PP			/+/				/+/
	MP		/+/	/+/		/+/		

Relationships between the pressure in the right atrium and the biochemistry of the cerebral blood outflow/inflow are presented in Tables 16-17.

Table 16.
Relationships between the pressure in RA and the biochemical parameters of the cerebral blood outflow

Group	RA	K pl	K er	Na pl	Na er	pH	pCO_2	SB	pO_2	HBO_2	HB	Ht	F-n	P-n	$AVDO_2$
N	A	/-/				/-/				/-/			/-/		/+/
	X	\-\	/-/						/-/	/-/	/-/	/+/	/-/		/-/
	V	/-/	/+/	/-/		/+/		/+/	/-/	/-/		/+/	/+/		/+/
	Y	/-/	/+/	/-/	/-/	/+/			/-/	/-/	/-/	/+/	/-/		/+/
	RA	K pl	K er	Na pl	Na er	pH	pCO_2	SB	pO_2	HBO_2	HB	Ht	F-n	P-n	$AVDO_2$
SAH	A														
	X			/+/			/+/								
	V								/+/						
	Y														

SAH patients demonstrate loss of the relationship between the pressure levels in RA and the values of general and plasma viscosity (F-n, Ht), vasoactive regulators of CVBF (Kl, K er, pH), and cerebral end metabolites (HbO_2,$AVDO_2$). The above data on relationships between pressure levels in SS, IJV, and RA (a single hemodynamic chamber with negative pressure differential) suggest that this zone can be seen as one of the regulators of cerebral gas exchange, where the main regulator is the minimum pressure along the path of the cerebral outflow—in RA. In SAH patients, this regulation channel is absent. In SAH patients, the relationships between the pressure levels in the zone regulating the cerebral gas exchange against the minimum pressure are lost or inverted for physical and chemical values of cerebral blood inflow, general and plasma viscosity (F-n, Ht), vasoactive ABC substances, and values of plasma and associated gases (pCo_2,HbO_2).

Table 17.

Relationships between the RA pressure levels and the biochemical parameters of the cerebral blood inflow

Group		K pl	K er	Na pl	Na er	pH	pCO_2	SB	pO_2	HBO_2	HB	Ht	F-n	P-n
N	A	/-/			/-/		/-/					/+/	/-/	
	X	/-/			/-/					/+/		/+/	\+\	
	V	/-/		/-/	/-/	/+/					/+/	/+/		
	Y	/-/		/-/	/-/	/+/	/-/			/+/		/+/	/-/	
		K pl	K er	Na pl	Na er	pH	pCO_2	SB	pO_2	HBO_2	HB	Ht	F-n	P-n
SAH	A								/-/				\+\	
	X			/+/	/-/	/-/			/-/					
	V			/+/					/-/					
	Y	/+/	/+/	/+/					/-/				/+/	

Summarizing the data given in the tables (18 and 19), we should point out that in SAH patients (when all Ao pressure values increase significantly) the relationship between the Ao levels and all values of the physical and chemical properties of the cerebral blood inflow and outflow (including values of plasma viscosity, membrane permeability, gas pressure, ABC) is lost or becomes inverted, while CBF, $AVDO_2$ and SinP levels remain comparable with the normal range.

The results that we obtained and processed by using methods of mathematical statistics, discussed in our publications [9], suggest that rheological properties of blood and viscosity can be seen as the initially regulated parameter of homeostasis in healthy people.

We assume, as proven, that the integrated hydrodynamic formation with a negative pressure differential—SinP–IJV–SVC–RA—is one of the cerebral gas exchange regulators, where the main regulator is the minimum pressure along the pathway of cerebral blood outflow : in the right atrium.

Table 18.
Relationships between the arterial pressure and the biochemical parameters of the cerebral blood inflow

Group		K pl	K er	Na pl	Na er	pH	pCO_2	SB	pO_2	HBO_2	HB	Ht	F-n	P-n
N	SP												/+/	
	DP						/-/	/-/					/+/	
	PP													
	MP						/-/	/-/	\+\					
SAH	SP									/+/	/-/			
	DP						/+/	/+/			/-/			
	PP													
	MP						/+/	/+/						

Table 19.
Relationships between the arterial pressure and the biochemical parameters of the cerebral blood outflow

Group		K pl	K er	Na pl	Na er	pH	pCO_2	SB	pO_2	HBO_2	HB	Ht	F-n	P-n
N	SP													
	DP			/+/									/+/	
	PP												/-/	
	MP			/+/				/-/						
SAH	SP			/-/							/-/			
	DP			/-/		/+/				/+/				
	PP				/-/						/-/		/+/	
	MP	/-/	/-/	/-/		/+/				/+/				

SAH is characterized by loss of homeostatic control of the factors determining rheological and thrombogenic properties of blood, which are involved in development of ischemic cerebral events. The regulation channel of cerebral gas exchange, which is represented by the minimum pressure along the pathway of the outflow from the brain, is also lost.

The results of the mathematical processing of the obtained source data are given in the above tables and can be used for a consolidated matrix table showing synergistic relationships between the groups of exchange and hemodynamics parameters participating in maintenance of homeostasis stability in healthy people.

Our arrangement of the results, which is given below, is a dynamic matrix norm (DMN) of relationships typical of the exchange and hemodynamics (the homeostasis balance mechanism) in healthy people. In the following publications we supplement DMN with the results of similar studies involving vascular systems of other organs (Table 20).

Table 20.

Dynamic homeostasis control matrix in healthy humans (in norm- DMN)

		Ao				RA					RV		LV				Sin P				BSBR				
		SP	DP	PP	MP	A	X	V	Y	MP	FDP	MP	SP	PP	CO	SV	SP	DP	PP	MP	K er	Ht	F-n	P-n	H-b
AO	K pl					-	-	-	-	X	X	X	X	X	X	X	+								-
	K er									X	X	X	X	X	X	X	-	-		-					
	Na pl							-	-	X	X	X	X	X	X	X	+	+			-	-	-	+	
	Na er					-	-	-	-	X	X	X	X	X	X	X	-				+				
	pH							+	+	X	X	X	X	X	X	X	-	-		-			+	-	+
	pCO2		-		-	-			-	X	X	X	X	X	X	X									
	SB		-		-					X	X	X	X	X	X	X	-	-		-					
	pO2				+					X	X	X	X	X	X	X	+	+		+	+		-	+	
	Hb O2						+		+	X	X	X	X	X	X	X								-	
	Hb							+		X	X	X	X	X	X	X	-	-		-		+	+	-	
	Ht					+	+	+	+	X	X	X	X	X	X	X	-	-		-			+	+	+
	F-n	+	+			-	+		-	X	X	X	X	X	X	X	-	-		-		+		+	+
	P-n									X	X	X	X	X	X	X	+	+		+			+		-
SinP	K pl					-	-	-	-	X	X	X	X	X	X	X	-	-		-			+		
	K er						-	+	+	X	X	X	X	X	X	X									
	Na pl		+		+			-	-	X	X	X	X	X	X	X	+	+		+	+	+		+	
	Na er								-	X	X	X	X	X	X	X					+				-
	pH					-		+	+	X	X	X	X	X	X	X	-	-		-	-	+			
	pCO2									X	X	X	X	X	X	X		+							
	SB				-			+		X	X	X	X	X	X	X	-	-		-			+		
	pO2						-	-	-	X	X	X	X	X	X	X					+				
	Hb O2					-	-	-	-	X	X	X	X	X	X	X								-	
	Hb						-		-	X	X	X	X	X	X	X	-	-		-					
	Ht						+	+	+	X	X	X	X	X	X	X								+	
	F-n		+	-		-	-	+	-	X	X	X	X	X	X	X	-	-		-				-	
	P-n									X	X	X	X	X	X	X	+			+			-		
	AVDO2	X	X	X	X	+	-	+	+	X	X	X	X	X	X	X		+		+	-			+	+
SinP	SP				+	-	+			+		+	-	-	-										
	DP		+		+		+			+		+	-	-	-										
	PP		-				-				+														
	MP				+		+		+	+	-	+	-	-	-	-									

Conclusion

The multitude of correlation relationships inherent in the examined parameters (which will be expended in the following publications) and represented in DMN demonstrates synergistic relationships among all studied elements of the homeostatic regulation in healthy people.

The sets of qualitative interrelationships of biochemical substances, which are shown in DMN, including relationships between hemodynamics, biochemistry and hemodynamics in reference points of the human body, make it possible to devise new (complementing the existing ones) methods and techniques of diagnosis, evaluation and adjustment of the entire range of health and disease conditions in humans.

The comparative analysis of any clinical or research data against DMN, as it was shown above by using the example of arterial hypertension, offers new diagnostic, pharmacological and experimental opportunities in clinical practice, experimental medicine, and biological sciences.

References

1. Auerr L. Pial arterial reactions to hyper- and hypocapnia: a dynamic experimental study in cats. Eur Neurol. 1978; 17(6);351-62.

2. Cameron JR, Caronna J. The effect of local changes in potassium and bicarbonate concentration on hypothalamic blood flow in the rabbit. J Physiol.1976;262(2):415-30.

3. Ernst E. Plasma fibrinogen--an independent cardiovascular risk factor.J Intern Med. 1990;227(6):365-72.

4. Kety SS. Cerebral circulation. In: Handbook of physioligy; Washington 1960 (5),1751.

5. Lassen NA, Christensen MS. Physiology of cerebral blood flow. Br J Anaesth. 1976;48(8):719-34.

6. Rossanda M, Sganzerla EP. Acid-base and gas tension on measurements in cerebrospinal fluid. Brit J Anaesth. 1976; 48(8):753-60.

7. Tranqui-Poit L, Marder VJ, Suscillon M, Budzynski AZ, Hurdly-Clergeon J. Electron microscopic studies of plasmic degradation products of fibrinogen. Implication for disulfide structure of fibrinogen. Biochem Biophys Acta. 1975; 400(2):189-99.

8. Guria GT Macroscopic structure formation in blood dynamics in the light of the theory of unbalanced structures. A dissertation for the degree of Doctor of Physical and Mathematical Sciences. Moscow State University, 2002.

9. Kruglov AG, Gebel GY, Vasilyev AY. Impact of intra-extracranial hemodynamics on cerebral ischemia by arterial hypertension (Part 1 and Part 2). Int I Biomed 2012; 2(2):89-101.

CHAPTER 2.

ARTERIOVENOUS RELATIONSHIP IN THE PATHOGENESIS OF ENCEPHALOPATHY

The study of the relationship of the intracranial venous pressure with systemic arterial pressure and central pressure in stabile arterial hypertension (SAH), compared to the equivalent part of DYNAMIC MATRIX OF THE NORM (DMN), is a main issue of this work. We built a model of the impact of the intracranial and cerebral blood flow on the development of disturbances in neuron activity and hypertonic angioencephalopathy (HAE) formation. Despite the importance of the problem, there are a small number of studies dedicated to impairments in the cerebral venous system in HAE. There is no consensus about the primary or secondary nature of venous pathology in arterial hypertension. Modem concepts of HAE pathogenesis mainly associate the clinical manifestations with the active processes in the arterial vascular bed. In particular, ischemic attack, "small" strokes, and progressive cerebral ischemia and considered as the main causes of HAE. There is a great deal of literature dedicated to changes in the structure and functions of intra- and extracerebral arteries and only a few studies dedicated to the role of the cerebral venous vascular bed in the development of HAE. In one such study, have found a brain venous hemodynamic abnormality with an increase in blood flow volume and decrease in venous velocity, as well as an increase of the linear velocity in the arterial flow [1].

The purpose of this study was to create a model of relationship between the intracranial/cerebral arterial and venous flows both among themselves and with the systemic arterial pressure and central pressure; create a concept of HAE pathogenesis, taking into account the abnormalities of the metabolic support for the actualized neural networks and related changes in the mental sphere.

For all participants, the study was conducted in the same laboratory by the same methods. Results are given in Chapter 1.

The results indicate the levels of intracranial venous (IVP) blood pressure in the cerebral sigmoid sinus (SS) and in the venous system of the brain (IJV) (Tabl. 1-2).

Table 1.
SinP levels (mmHg)

Group		SP	DP	PP	MP
N	M	10.5	8.3	2.4	9.4
	m	2.2	1.8	0.75	2.2
	Max	21	16.8	4.2	18.9
	Min	6	3.9	0.5	4.9
SAH	M	11.5	7.7	3.8	10.1
	m	3.2	2.9	1.4	3.9
	Max	22.6	19.2	7	20.4
	Min	3.9	2.1	1.3	2.4

Table 2.
Pressure levels (mmHg) in IJV

Group		SP	DP	PP	MP
N	M	7.3	5.5	2.1	6.7
	m	1.1	1	0.6	1.3
	Max	13.8	10.5	5.1	11.7
	Min	2.4	2	0.2	1.4
SAH	M	8.7	6.3	2.6	7.2
	m	3.4	3.3	1.1	3.2
	Max	21	14	6.4	15.7
	Min	2.4	0.5	1.2	2.1

For intracranial venous pressure (SinP) we note despite being within the boundaries of the “zone of norm,” a reliable growth of pressure level (by 8% to 9%), especially significant for the pulse pressure (by 58%). Presence of the pressure gradient between the intra- and extracranial venous systems, despite the varying levels of pressure in the IJV (the effect of intrathoracic and barometric pressure), proves that IVP is formed with the participation of the factors affecting in IJV. Previously [2,3] we have observed a radical change in the composition and quality of the correlations for intra- and extracranial blood flow with other parameters in SAH. Particularly important are the loss or inversion of correlations with the parameters of general and plasma viscosity and rheology, as well as the loss of correlations with the final gas exchange products of the brain that determine the plasma gas tension (O_2, CO_2).

All levels of pressure in the right atrium (RA) in SAH (out MP) significantly exceed the boundaries of the normal zone (Table 3). Pressure levels in Ao and LV are shown in Table 4.

Table 3.
Pressure levels (mmHg) in RA and RV

Group		RA					RV	
		A	X	V	Y	P	EDP	MP
N	M	5.7	2.4	4.6	3.4	4.1	5.1	14.4
	m	0.9	0.7	0.8	0.2	1.1	1.2	1.8
	Max	8.8	5.3	6.5	6.0	8.4	10	19.8
	Min	3.0	0	1.6	0	1.2	0	8.8
SAH	M	7.4	4.0	6.4	4.7	3.4	3.4	13.9
	m	2.7	2.1	2.8	2.0	2.6	2.6	4.4
	Max	11.8	9.0	14.1	9.0	8.4	8.4	28
	Min	1.8	0	1.8	0	0	0	6.6

Table 4.
Pressure levels (mmHg) in Ao and LV

Group		CO	SV	Ao				LV	
				SP	DP	PP	MP	SP	PP
N	M	10.9	128.4	114	71	40.3	92.6	108	100.5
	m	1.3	22.4	4.5	3.8	3.5	5.1	6.4	7.1
	Max	18.7	186	147	87	65	115	130	130
	Min	5.5	80	90	50	21	70	90	85
SAH	M	11.1	147	180	101	79	137	180	168
	m	3.1	38.9	31	21	22	23	34	28
	Max	21.7	246	270	155	144	210	260	248
	Min	5.3	50	150	78	40	96	150	138

Previously, we analyzed correlations between parameters of RA pressure and indicators of SinP as well as between the biochemical parameters (including rheological parameters) of blood flowing from the brain [3]. We found a loss of correlations for pressure among the parameters of general and plasma viscosity, vasoactive regulators of cerebral blood flow (electrolytes), and final metabolites of the brain (arteriovenous difference in O_2 and HbO_2) in H. In other word, during development of SAH there is a loss of regulatory relationships of the RA and SinP with brains metabolites and metabolites and rheological parameters in a single hemodynamical chamber (IVP-RA), where the main regulator, in our opinion, is the minimal pressure in the outflow tract from the brain: in the RA: The data in the

Table 4 are well known and shown for complete characterization of the study issue. In norm, the active process of the left ventricle (LV) systole (systolic and pulse pressure in aorta (Ao) and LV) have no correlations with the pulse pressure (PP) in SinP (Table 5). LV systolic and pulse pressures are in negative association with systolic, diastolic and mean pressure of SinP. Consequently, the formation of IVP in norm does not depend on Ao PP, at the same time it has a relationship with the systolic, diastolic and mean pressure in Ao. In H, there is a loss of the correlation between SinP and the pressure in the aortic chamber, but a correlation between the active phase of LV and PP is found. Thus, in norm SinP levels correlate with the LV ejection phase; maximum of pressure in system SinP--Ao is achieved with opening of the aortic valve; maximal pressure for the skull (brain) is formed; a wave process in Ao (immediate application area is extra- and intracranial blood vessels) is generated.

Table 5.
Correlations between SinP and Ao - LV

Group	SinP	Ao				CO	LV	
		SP	DP	PP	MP		SP	PP
N	SP				+	-	-	-
	DP		+		+	-	-	-
	PP		-					
	MP				+	-	-	-
SAH	SP			+				
	DP							
	PP	+	+	+	+		+	
	MP	-	-		-			

In the horizontal position, LV systole, forming a rotational and translational movement around the outer (variable) axis in the form of a spherical wave structure [4] of aortic flow, reaches all areas of the body before closing the aortic valve [5]. The negative correlation with the levels of SinP is explained only by the existence of a characteristic structure between the cavity of the skull and extracranial vessels, which changes its clearance under the influence of the wave process. We believe that this structure is carotid artery siphons (CASs) located in the cavernous sinus. CASs are guides for wave structures of the heart; they are informative characteristics of different levels of regulation [2] interfering in the cavernous sinuses of the dura mater. The presence of CASs explains the negative relations between the SinP and LV ejection phase in norm. This relation changes diametrically in SAH and becomes positive, which indicates parallel changes in SinP and Ao pressure, which are possible only as a result of changes of functional relationships the system CASs-cavernous sinus which is connected through the *sinus petrosi inferior* with the zone of catheter wedging while obtaining the initial data. It should be also noted that the sympathetic plexus of CASs participates in innervations of the eyeball, which plays an important role in purposeful behavior. The increased IVP in SAH is necessary to maintain the pressure gradient at the required level to ensure the adequate perfusion and cerebral metabolic processes (in the zone of norm). This is possible only if the ability to the extracranial regulation (the defeated CASs) is lost, as well as the lesion of the intracranial vascular bed with narrowing of the lumen and rigidity of vascular wall.

We consider the phase of aortic peak during Ao and LV separation as 1) a final stage of the high-energy phase and 2) an initial stage of the diastolic evolution. The action of CASs, whose contraction is caused by LV systole, makes a "selection" (damping) of the pressure, starting with a value equal to the average BP. Pressure levels exceeding the average BP in norm remain in "reserve" to respond in stressful situations (in principle, it is quite a minimal adaptive response, namely, the diminution of CAS reaction to the aortic wave process). First of all, the average BP is positively associated with SinP up to diastolic BP, which indicates the setting of the unified hydrodynamic system (Ao - vessels entering the skull - SinP) in the phase of the diastolic evolution (from average to diastolic pressure). This explains the positive relationship of the diastolic evolution of the intracranial venous bed with the aortic diastolic evolution. Achieving minimal values by the Ao-SinP gradient is replaced by the LV systole. In other words, Ao pressure--SinP relationships change their own correlation from the negative through "zero" to the positive (during the cardiac cycle). The radical difference for SAH is: 1) the dependence of SinP only on the high-energy phase with an inversion of direction of regulation; 2) the lack of correlation at all stages of the diastolic evolution; 3) the lack of a reserve of pressure for urgent adaptation. Thus, during H development, despite the increase in energy expenditure to ensure the cerebral blood flow and metabolism, the efficiency of metabolic support for the brain functioning is reduced. Our data [2] suggest that during SAH development, there is a loss of the hemodynamic mechanisms for correction of the negative manifestations of hyperfibrinogenemia, rheological and viscous blood parameters, and thrombus formation; ie, there is a loss of regulation of conjugation between thrombotic factors and pressure towards the outflow from the brain, both of which exist in norm. Pathways of the venous outflow according to the pressure gradient from the cortex through the venous sinuses in the RA have no valves, making a unified hemodynamic chamber [2]. The pressure at the outlet of the intracerebral venous bed in the zone of minimal pressure significantly increases the entire range of values in SAH. The critical value for intravascular pressure in veins depends on the ratio of wall thickness to the radius of the vessel and elastic modulus. Loss of stability and a sharp change in the lumen of the intracranial veins occurs at pressure changes by 0.2 to 0.5 mmHg resulting in a change in the throughput volume capability and the cross-sectional shapes of venules and veins. A gradient of transmural pressure effects in the system "liquor-veins" is possible in both directions, and an increase in venous pressure, causing the maximal volume flow, increases the transmission pressure on the liquor. The decreased venous blood flow, which is accompanied by liquor hypertension, is found in SAH. The increase in venous stasis is a marker of decompensation of cerebral circulation. A disparity between the rate of arterial inflow and venous return (delay) is more pronounced in patients with chronic heart failure [6]. We believe that in a unified hydrodynamic chamber with the outflow according to the pressure gradient, the disturbances in any portion of unified hemodynamic space "intracerebral veins—RA" [2] affect the condition and regulation of the entire intra- and extracerebral venous flow regardless of the exposure vector (along or against the blood flow). Increasing the "booster" venous pressure in the valveless bloodstream inevitably leads to increased pressure in the main outflow tracts from the brain (1: superior sagittal sinus - bridging veins - cortical cuff - cortical veins; 2: straight sinus - deep cerebral veins -cortical veins) against the blood flow to the functional unit of the micro vasculature network: post-capillary venule—capillary— pre-capillary arterioles. The increase in the "booster" venous pressure according to the previously described mechanism [3] is spread through valveless veins on the entire volume of the brain, and affects the liquor pressure in accordance with the transfer mechanism.

The minimum dimensions of the neural structures, in which there are the marked changes in blood flow (functional hyperemia—FH) under functional load, correspond to the size of neural columns. According to G. Mchedlishvili [7], the initial stage of FH has neurogenic regulation, but the K/Na pump having the mechanisms of metabolic supply for neurons has almost the same time parameters. During development of the activity in the exchange field of the actualized neural network (the excited neurons), the venous vessels eliminating metabolites are already in a state of maximum volumetric capacity without the possibility to remove the additional blood volume by changing the volume of the venous vessels.

The decreased rate of blood flow in the micro vasculature cannot be compensated for by a Fareusa-Lindqvist effect. Additional complicating factors of blood flow in the macro- and microcirculation networks are disorders in aggregation, rheology and viscosity properties of blood with the loss of homeostatic control, and loss of regulation of the hemodynamic and biochemical interactions, which take place in norm [2]. All of this results in a delay in metabolite elimination, 0_2 deficiency, an excess of $C0_2$, a lack of glucose, changes in intra- and extravascular concentration of electrolytes (regardless of the activity of transmembrane channels), increased platelet activity, and other abnormal reactions (i.e, all of the above are indicators of the development of local circulatory hypoxia). Disturbances in the metabolism of neurons, which occur due to the lack of substrates for oxidation, lead to a reduced formation of macroergic substances (ATP, ADP, creatine phosphate). Accumulation of metabolites is a disturbing factor. Thus, with an increase in the activity of neurons and formation of activated neural associations, there is a local circulatory hypoxia. Manifestations of circulatory hypoxia are the changes in activity of selective channels of membranes, and in their permeability (especially for Na, K, and Ca) and excitability, and destruction of structural patterns of neurons (nucleus, organelles, and cytoplasm). The excess of the oxidized metabolites plays a special role in damaging cellular and intracellular membranes. A result of this excess is characterized by the development and progression of degenerative processes in neurons, impaired intracellular signaling (both in neurons and the adjustable effector cells), a change of phosphorylation and the activity of functional proteins. Many researchers characterize the disturbances in the energy supply of K/Na, Ca membrane pumps leading to abnormalities in the transmembrane gradient of electrolyte concentrations as one of the main mechanisms of neuronal hypoxia. These disturbances lead to membrane depolarization and inactivation of the transmembrane channels. Abnormalities in the calcium pump reduce Ca release from cytosol to the extracellular environment with deposition in endoplasmic reticulum. There is a reduction of FH in the projection area of the conditioned response caused by a decrease in the blood supply to the cortex in SAH [8].

The total result of the above-described is a disturbance of the integrative activity of the nervous system in different forms: the pathological determinants, the pathological dominants, the pathological systems and others [9], as well as the suppression of neuronal population activity [10].

In hypoxic changes of cortex, hyperexcitability (a decreased threshold) and metabolic acidosis, the sensory stimulus for activation and the subsequent activity of neural networks have a lower (compared with the norm) power and duration of the signal for initiating the operation of the "answer" mechanism and metabolic supply for the exchange fields of the involved neurons. The reduced energy level of the initial signal means an increase in the total amount of information and the range of the readable signals from the environment.

The increase in size of the information field and excessive sensory stimulation (as a consequence) associated with difficulty in selecting the main control signal leads to excessive stimulation of the synapses of the afferent impulses and changes in the efficiency of synaptic transmission in the form of long-term potentiation and depression (pathological excitation or inhibition). Abnormalities in the allocation of the main control signals lead to the deficit model of reality distortion and the disturbance of translational symmetry. Formation of an objective reality model having an information deficit and mismatch leads to discrepancies in the projection mechanisms to the real parameters of the environment, as well as disturbances of the adequacy and determinism in the system "environment - man - environment." Projection is a way of interacting, adapting, and searching for methods to maintain homeostatic equilibrium ("Deterministic equivalent response" according to Le Chatelier). Having a structural mismatch to the original information field (objective reality) the "projection" (cognitive product) is not equivalent, but rather asymmetric, to the content of the external world, with a growing parametric discrepancy. The consequence of this is: an increasing mismatch in stimulus-response; stereotyping of behavioral forms (the result of the stable existence of neural associations of standard answer); a decrease in the adaptive arsenal; and adjustment disorder (physiological, psychological, and social).

Conclusion

There is a loss of homeostatic control for the hemodynamic, (extra- and intracerebral) and biochemical regulation in SAH; the damping function of carotid siphons is impaired; the high-energy processes of the aortic chamber (systolic and pulse pressure) spread to the bloodstream of the brain; cerebral venous stasis is formed; increased pressure in the microvascular network of the brain is defined; and a loss of the homeostatic control of the rheological properties of blood is defined. The loss of extracranial regulation of intracranial venous pressure in SAH leads to venous plethora of the intracerebral vessels, increasing the "booster" pressure in the microvasculature, and circulatory hypoxia of brain tissues. The consequences of these changes are metabolic and hemodynamic disturbances in energy supply for activated neurons, as well as circulatory hypoxia resulting in disturbances of the regulatory function of the nervous system and mental activity, and the development of HAE.

References

1. Machin VV, Belova LA, Belov VG, Salikhova EA. Cerebral discirculation in arterial hypertension (clinical and ultrasound). Klin Fiziol Krov. 2009; 1:40-4.
2. Kruglov A, Gebel G, Vasilyev A. Intracranial venous pressure as possible determinant of mental regulation. Int J Biomed. 2011;l(4):245-8.
3. Kruglov A, Gebel G, Vasilyev A. Impact of intra - extracranial hemodynamics on cerebral ischemia by arterial hypertension (Part 1-2). Int J Biomed. 2012;2(2):89-102.
4. Kuzmina NB, Drogaicev AD. Formation of blood flow in the cavity of the left ventricle. In book: Cardiac physiology. Series: Manual of physiology; 1980:212-4.
5. Lightfoot A. Transport phenomena in live systems. Biomedical aspects of momentum and mass transport. M.: Mir, 1977.
6. Zolotukhina NS. Hypertensive encephalopathy: venous brain discirculation in patients with chronic heart failure. Abstract of PhD Thesis. Moscow; 2006
7. Mchedlishvili GI. Microcirculation. M.: Nauka; 1989:203-204.
8. Khananashvili YaA. Blood supply of the cerebral cortex and its bioelectric activity in the dynamics of arterial hypertension. Abstract of ScD Thesis. Leningrad; 1990.
9. Kryzhanovsky GN. Discirculatory pathology of the nervous system. Moscow: MedInform Agentstvo; 2009.
10. Levin SG, Shamsudinov AA, Goduhin OV. Comparative effect of blockers of ATP-sensitive K+ -channels on the induced changes in activity of pyramidal neurons of hippocampal area CA1 under brief episodes of hypoxia. Bull Exp Biol Med. 2012; 10:435-8.

CHAPTER 3.

INTRACRANIAL VENOUS PRESSURE AS A POSSIBLE PARTICIPANT IN DETERMINATION OF MENTAL REGULATION

Mechanisms of intracranial pressure (ICP) formation in humans and their dependence on arterial (BP), venous (VP), capillary and liquor (LP) pressures have been studied for many decades. The influence of factors determining the level and fluctuations in ICP is limited to the change of ratio between the volumes of the components occupying the cranial cavity. Changes of their total volume cause shifts of LP. Liquor is the transmission link between arterial vessels, venous vessels and the elements of brain tissue. CVBF, which provides adequate brain activity, is changed only when LP exceeds VP, after which CVBF is reduced proportionally to the rise in BP, causing violations of the brain activity.

Regarding the regulation of cerebral venous blood flow, opinions differ, from denying the influence of venous blood flow on CVBF in normal conditions to suggesting the prevalence of neural influences serving the system requirements, or the dependence on blood flow in the exchange field of the brain, among others. Several authors [1-3] experimentally confirmed the dependence of cerebral circulation on venous circulation, highlighting the uncertainty of regulatory mechanisms of these processes.

A. Shidlovsky et al. in 1979 [4] experimentally confirmed the data obtained from the model and showed that the most effective effector link is venous elasticity, causing the greatest change of functions in three subsystems: arterial reservoir, heart, and venous system. The range of views of researchers on the relationship between pressures (VP-LP) in the brain tissue is narrow: from full compliance of LP and VPs to excessive VP in the brain veins in relation to LP, but with a lower level of VP in the brain sinuses. It has been shown that the critical value of VP depends on the ratio of wall thickness to the radius of the vessel and the modulus of elasticity of the wall [5]. Even with a small predominance of external over internal pressure (0.2- 0.5 mmHg), stability of the veins is lost, and their lumen changes abruptly. An increase in ICP causes transformation of intracerebral vein lumen from circular to oval-shaped, and then to a slit-like shape. With rising ICP and the excessive VP, the vessel is collapsed, the inner lumen of a vein is closed, followed by cessation of venous flow in the microcirculatory bed and the oppression of metabolism in the brain tissues.

In the concept presented, the venous blood flow in the brain tissue is regarded as a hemodynamic, bio-physical component of the interdependent, synergistic mechanisms of mental activity that provide the functional associations between neural networks and metabolic supply to activated neurons. Note that the cell bodies of neurons, occupying about 5% of the cerebral cortex, consume 25% of all the oxygen supply, which must be covered by an adequate volume of CVBF as early as in the first phase of functional hyperemia. Excited neurons with subsequent transition to an active state of elements, united in a functional circuit, require metabolic processes; an increase in the volume of inflowing blood, which happens only due to changes in the inner lumen of the cortical artery with no possibility of changing its outside diameter, would lead to compression of elements surrounding the brain tissue. Note that the amplitude of the lumen in cortical arteries increases as their caliber decreases. Volumetric blood flow in the smaller size vessels is also increased due to the Fahraeus-Lindquist effect, lowering blood viscosity. Microcirculation increases due to the transition of plasma capillaries to a state allowing an increased number of active capillaries. There are four regulatory circuits of CVBF—neurogenic, humoral, metabolic, and myogenic—and priority is given to the circuit most suited to the situation.

Purpose of this part of the work: definition of the theory model with regard to the interrelation of CVBF in the microcirculatory bloodstream and initiation of psychic regulation in humans under normal conditions. The subject of the study was the hemodynamic and biophysical equivalent of metabolic supply of activated neural circuits, i.e. initiated and lasting mental activity.

Postcapillary venules and brain veins are a special interest in the proposed concept as they have a central place in the scheme, uniting the effector component of mental activity and hemodynamic gradient (vector of ratio of LP to VP). Parameters of VP and CSF pressure are well known and have no significance for our study. The main subject of discussion is the dynamics of gradient venous relations between two liquid media, that is, human intracerebral venous blood and liquor fluid under normal conditions, in the context of neural network activity onset and metabolic provision.

Brain veins have a thin wall consisting of 1 to 2 layers of endothelium and a connective tissue layer without elastic and muscular plexus.

It seems that the intracerebral veins normally can operate in two states:

1. When neurons in the metabolic field served are activated (maximum blood supply): intravascular pressure is higher than LP, section of vein is circular;

2. In resting neurons, with a minimum metabolic level, intravascular pressure is equal to LP, section of vein is oval, slit.

Thus, if any activity occurs in the metabolic field, i.g., during excitation of neurons in the averting vessel, even in the first phase of functional hyperemia, due to the increased volume of local blood flow, intravascular pressure increases. The vein, increasing in volume, takes a cylindrical shape, reaching its maximum permeability (with a circular cross section).

Intracranial space is closed for fast processes (initiated in less than one cardiac cycle) due to hydraulic resistance to redistribution of fluid volumes [6]. At the same time, in the intracranial space a balance exists among the amount of brain substance, of cerebrospinal fluid, and of blood [6,7].

Excessive pressure of the **intracerebral veins**, which increase in volume, spreads through the cerebrospinal fluid spherically along the activated neural circuit and can be utilized in the incompressible, non-displaced space by only one structure, intracerebral veins, which are not involved in the metabolic supply of the activated neural circuit. For the period of excess LP the transmural pressure from outside the wall of uninvolved veins increases, with an increase of intravascular pressure and compensatory outflow by the pressure gradient and change in cross section of the vein (oval, slit-like shape), and with a decrease of the **volume** capacity, thereby retaining VP increases in the functional microvasculature unit (backwards): vein —> postcapillary venule —> capillary —> precapillary arteriole —> arteriole. Therefore, integration of the mechanisms for the metabolic securing of initiation of the neurons involved in other non-activated neural associations is complicated. Thus, the hemodynamic biophysical gradient effect of the actualized neural circuit in the attainable radius of influence leads to difficulty in initiating the metabolic securing of non-activated neural circuits, creating a competitive environment, and increasing the threshold of neuron excitability. At the same time, the vascular network, with maximal volume of blood flow due to the lasting activity of the neural circuit, causes excessive pressure and is less vulnerable to external pressor effects. Perhaps this is the hemodynamic equivalent of reverberation and other continuing conditions, as well as of neural structures that ensure vital functions. We believe that the first stages of initiated mental activity in the brain tissue, realized by actualized neural circuits, develop the biophysical phenomenon of excessive pressure (non-pulsating, non¬cardiac) as a wave dissipative structure, spherically spreading through the liquor fluid. It is creating a priority energy supply of activated neural circuits, counteracting other initiations, interfering with the wave consequences of active neural structures with sufficient energy supply.

The activity of neurons reflects their involvement in a system with the organization of all processes as the informational equivalent of the result, i.e. of the future event [8], where the mental factor acts as a systemic quality of the organization of physiological processes. Thus, the activity of neurons in the behavioral act system means that the behavior contains the mental activity, i.e., informational, determination of the physiological mechanisms through system processes. During the behavioral act, which has a hierarchical, gradient structure (for example, the implementation of a **need** as the most significant of the dispositions that supports purposeful activity to meet the need), the mental activity serves as a determinant of initiation and lasting activity of neural circuits, which in turn is a determinant of metabolic processes, determining the volumetric hemodynamic phenomenon, which is an antagonist of other initiations at the time (that is a measure of the relevance of motive) of the behavioral act's existence. It should be emphasized that the cooperative regulation of the functional system described acts in a series of deterministic gradient subsystems: **psyche —> neural associations —> exchange field, metabolism —> increased volume of CBF —> overpressure —> psyche**, where deactualization of a motive ceases the activity of the effector mechanisms.

Motive, as a stable property of the subject, a motive force, the reason for his behavior, is a set of dispositions, the most important of which is a **need** [8]. Need is considered as a state of dissatisfaction of the body (the person), lack of what is required to maintain a state of homeostatic equilibrium of the body. A feature of a live being is a selective character of response to the subject of actual **need**, to address the imbalance, i.e. to eliminate the gradient between the present state and the target state. The result for which the activity is undertaken is defined as the purpose, the mental image of the future result, formed by the subject, and is a major part of a deliberate regulatory process.

The goal, which is the mental image, possesses the characteristics of the model and, being a perceived determinant of behavior, forms the entire process of self-regulation as a vector with a difference of model parameters between the initial (present) and final (target) phases.

We create relations medium-individual under conditions of interoceptive fixation of metabolic psychological deviation, misbalance, followed by inclusion of homeostatic, behavioral correction as a state when the goal (future) state is more preferable than the present one. That is the difference between the present and the future states; whatever that difference is represented through (Na blood plasma concentration or stages of career path) defines the values of the goal state and its achievement vector. This very difference between the values of the goal and the present states of a subject that initiates homeostatic correction is identified as the "**motivation gradient**" (MG). It initiates and actualizes goal-oriented behavior. The end goal is to achieve the parametric equalization, i.e. elimination of the motivational gradient. Thus, MG stimulates the body (the person) to find the needed object to correct the imbalance, to restore the homeostatic equilibrium, i.e. to eliminate MG. Since imbalance, frustration and other forms of deficit, i.e. gradient states, in humans may occur across the full spectrum of needs (physical, spiritual, social, etc.), it is possible to use the term MG in its broadest application, both in physiology and in human psychology.

Considering homeostasis as the constancy of the parameters of the internal environment while the parameters of the environment are changed, the organism is regarded as a self-regulating system that tends to maintain a state of current balance, for physiological as well as for psychological parameters.

Targeted behavioral acts of any complexity and duration that are aimed to meet the actualized **need**, that is, to remove MG, have a hierarchical gradient structure and determine initiation and lasting activity of neural circuits; the discussed hemodynamic, biophysical gradient of the cerebral venous bed is the equivalent of their activity. Thus, MG, which has model characteristics in the form of a gradient of parameters of correlative - correlated operational patterns, has a consistent hemodynamic gradient (VP - LP in brain tissue) of actualized neural circuits that have morpho-physiological characteristics. The hemodynamic gradient emergence mechanism we described, irrespective of localization, is not available for invasive study techniques, which we have been applying in cerebral probing of humans. We believe that our theory can be verified by means of a functional MRI. There have been no materials related to this subject found in the available reading matter.

Initiation and duration of the existence of MG and equivalent hemodynamic gradient are determined by actualization of the motive and by achievement of the target state through purposeful behavior. Considering MG as a characteristic that indicates the direction of steepest change in the scalar variables, whose value varies from one point in space to another, we define the zero (starting) point of subjective time (ST) for the image of the target, which can be taken in psychological time as an abstract point, while the present is always a certain time interval [9] (in contrast to Husserl, who determined the zero point of ST at the stage: Now, currently). That image of the target is the psycho-physiological stimulus for MG formation and the starting point for the formation of an interim assessment scale for the rate of result achievement (ST). In pursuit of the goal, forward movement on MG thus means movement along the descending ST (time perspective) to the mark 0. Thus, we can assume that decreasing ST flow (the initiation, duration and staged rate of which are determined by the relevance of motive and by motivation) has a vector that is opposite to the vectors of MG and of increasing quantities (physical, biological) of time, reaching a zero value at the point of parametric equalization of MG.

In the sequence described, ST flow is only possible if some events occur in the subjective world (whose nature is irrelevant: perceptual, motor, cognitive events). The dependence of subjective length of time, from occupancy (subjectively shorter) to non-occupancy (subjectively long), on events has been experimentally confirmed: for example, consider the 5-fold excess density of ST in a 10-year-old child, compared to that of a 60-year-old man. Let us directly correlate the subjective sensation of speed of living life (time flow) with the total number of subjective events (density, saturation). As the subject gets older, he accumulates automated skills and fills the memory resources, and he creates, in addition to many short-term, often stereotyped tactical aims, several forward-looking plans for achieving long-term strategic aims, covering large time intervals. The structure of MG and ST for strategic purposes (as opposed to tactical ones) is discrete in the sense that the phenomena that are accompanied by changes of parameters may occur at periods separated by time intervals, while being in the narrative-directed sequence of events.

When one reaches a strategic target, ST is reset, with parametric equalization that means the end of the motivation that initiated MG, which is retrospectively perceived as a fused experienced event, regardless of the time actually lived. Motivational incentives in terms of strategic planning, forming the corresponding targets (images), determine the ST flow for a considerable length of time in discrete conditions; therefore, the current ST (filled largely by automated stereotypical actions) is perceived as less filled, slowed, while the goal, zeroing of ST, is subjectively experienced as quickly reached and tactical. We believe that the retrospective assessment of ST speed is subjectively quantized by event-driven narratives, smoothing the real times of achieving tactical and strategic purposes.

Conclusion

Initiation and duration of the existence of MG and the equivalent hemodynamics gradient are determined by actualization of the motive and by achievement of the target state through purposeful behavior. The lifetime (from the beginning to the disappearance) of an MG creates a subjective feeling of movement of ST. There is no prolonged state of stable present for a subject. Motivated by variable goal images due to metabolic and psychic deviations, misbalance, the subject is persistently in the vector space of motivational gradients of goals achieved one by one. The goals' images (the future) actualize the subject's adaptation dynamics. The present represents only a temporary pretension and is manifested by emotional connotations (+, 0, -) depending on matching-mismatching of the subject's actual state with the estimated waiting for parametric equalization, the state of homeostatic balance.

References

1. Labory A. Regulation of metabolic processes. Moscow: Medicine, 1980, 382 p. Moskalenko YE, Weinstein HB. The role of intracranial veins in the cerebral blood flow regulation mechanism. In: Proceeds of the international symposium on the regulation of capacitative vessels. Moscow: Medicine; 1977:120-129.
2. Moskalenko YE, Weinstein HB. The role of intracranial veins in the cerebral blood flow regulation mechanism. In: Proceeds of the international symposium on the regulation of capacitative vessels. Moscow: Medicine; 1977:120-129.
3. Tkachenko BI. Venous circulation. Leningrad; 1979.
4. Shidlovsky VA, Vezloyaschev DV, Lischuk VA, Ledenev VI, Nelyudova IV, Sadoyan DG. Biophysical properties of an isolated cardiovascular system. Krovoobraschenije. 1976; 5:29-36.
5. Moskalenko YE. Functional stability of the cerebral circulation. Physiological Journal. 1978; 64:589-97.
6. Moskalenko YE , Weinstein GB, Demchenko IT, Kislyakov YY, Krivchenko AI. Intracranial hemodynamics. Leningrad: Nauka; 1975:35-64.
7. Lerman VP. Cerebral circulatory disorders in intracranial tumors. Minsk; 1976.
8. Shvyrkov VB. Introduction to objective psychology. Neural basis of psychology. Moscow: Moscow Institute of Psychology of RAS; 1995.
9. Rubinstein SL. Fundamentals of General Psychology. Saint Petersburg: Piter; 2003.

CHAPTER 4.

MATHEMATICAL APPROACHES TO STUDYING THE IDEAL IMAGE OF THE GOAL

Modern theories in psychology and neurobiology, including principles and methods of experimental simulation and mathematical modeling of goal-directed behavior (GDB) and the approaches offered in computer-assisted instruction, lack completeness of perception and a clear description of "ideal" in the structure of GDB. The theories focus on the analysis of the environment and hierarchy of goals, neural network agents, systemogenesis of neural network structures and their mathematical models, and qualities of "intelligent agents" [1], etc. The core component of the integrated behavioral unit, the ideal image of the goal (IG) is, in our opinion, poorly interpreted in modem psychology and neurobiology.

Although we cannot furnish the IG mathematical models we are working on now in this publication, our desire is to introduce to you some of the mathematical methods that can help to create an adaptive model of the ideal portion of the behavioral unit (BU) (a metamer of behavioral continuum): viz., the ideal IG.

Discussion

According to P.K.Anokhin [2], integrated BU in the theory of functional systems of the second type, which supports the view that homeostasis, triggered by a change in behavior, is responsible for creating, retaining and subsequently removing the ideal IG, "a space-time structure" [3] in the activated neural circuits of the brain. Our concept is that the afferent part of BU is triggered by a significant imbalance in the parameter/parameters of the metabolic, psychological and social spectra, i.e. a departure from the bounds of the "normal zone." For metabolism, a deviation from the upper/lower bounds of the normal zone to the level of the suprathreshold sensitivity of the receptors is involved; for structures of the psychological and social spectra, involvement is to the level of "cognized–not-cognized" and "acceptable–not-acceptable." The distinguishing characteristic of "living beings" is their responsiveness to any disturbance in the homeostatic balance, to outright imbalance, i.e. the selective response to the object of an actual need. The need, being the most significant disposition of the motive, constitutes "an impelling force, a cause of the behavior" [4], which initiates the BU activation.

The normal zone is assumed to be the aggregate of the steady performance parameters, and is created by the confidence interval boundaries, where the probability of occurrence of another parameter value is >95%. The actual data on the average values, boundaries of the confidence interval, and relationships of the basic parameters of metabolism in healthy people, obtained using the probing method for arterial and venous blood, were reported in our prior publications [5].

The methods currently available can be applied only to the assumed equivalents of BU. It is, therefore, assumed that at the physiological level the BU core mechanism, involving the development of an acceptor of action results, i.e. IG creation and retention, is represented by an excitation circulating in a ring of interneurons [3]. We assume that the afferent information flow initiated by the homeostatic imbalance, is the ideal IG, which is synthesized and retained until the results are achieved; MG is a closed circular electrodynamic structure (EDS)generated by activated neuron networks [6].

Thus, IG is generated by an activated neural circuit functioning until the actualization of the effector part of BU is completed, until parametric equalization is reached, afference ceases and the parameter/parameters that actually caused the imbalance in the system is/are within the "normal zone".

IG, which we perceive at the current level of understanding, is a one-dimensional, time-extended creation, an integral characteristic of the individual who stays invariably in the vector space of alternately formed goals (in simplified form) and passes through the main stages of afference, creation of the ideal IG, efference, and reverse afference [2,3].

For the purpose of the systems analysis of the dynamics of adaptive self-regulation, it is feasible to employ an integrating term covering the IG "creation-retention" stage and the entire effector structure of BU: the motivational gradient (MG), where tIG=tMG.

We have best defined MG as an active distributed system (ADS) capable of spontaneously creating, in response to the information contained in IG, static and spatially heterogeneous structures facilitating adaptive behavior (for example, morphogenesis in a fertilized egg). ADS behavior types are described by non-linear differential equations [7].

As MG reveals model characteristics of a future result and acts as the determinant of behavior, it establishes the mechanism and the vector of the self-regulation process resulting from GDB producing parametric equalization, need satisfaction and motive removal. We present an equivalent MG, a hemodynamic, scalar gradient (with morphophysiological characteristics) as MG biophysical "marker" (with the dynamics of the characteristics inherent in "correlated-correlating operating images"): venous-liquor pressure in the exchange field of actualized neural circuits [8].

Perceiving MG as the route of the fastest change in the scalar values that are changing from one space point to another, we define the zero (starting) point of ST required in the IG structure for the expected action result (EAR), which in psychological time can be assumed as an abstract point, while "the present is always a certain interval" [9]. EAR is a constructive outcome of the ideal IG. The action result (AR) itself is the final stage of GDB that is effected through MG discontinuing the BU afference at the point of parametric equalization. The occurrence of EAR is the starting point of constructing an assessment scale of the time required to achieve the result. During the goal-achieving process, the linear motion from MG to the AR implies the decreasing motion of ST (to the "0" point in EAR). In other words, the decreasing time flow involves a vector which is opposite to the vectors of the effector part of MG with increasing values of (physical, biological) time, reaching the "zero" value at the point of parametric equalization. Therefore, the ST flow can exist only if events do exist in the inward world of an individual, irrespective of their nature or type. Thus, being a one-dimensional structure, possessing a duration value (tST =tIG = tMG) and a vector, ST can also find use as a vector "marker" of IG (MG).

Goal formation (voluntary/involuntary, actualized/ latent, strategic/ interim) can be described as the "behavioral continuum of alternately changing components" [4]: BUs "flowing" from the "previous" into the "next" (with the possibility of different sequence options, including transformation, "overlapping", interference, etc.).. The intervals between BU actualizations depend on variations in the homeostasis parameters prior to reaching the suprathreshold level and an initiation of the subsequent (latent) IG.

It is our understanding that goal formation determined by the imbalanced system is a continuous representation from one space-objective reality to another,- space-mental structures of representation (with different dimensional, time, space, etc., categories) and the subsequent projection of the mental structures into the external world through GDB. Thus, the correlation between sets is established, where near points of the evaluation develop into near points of the values. In the information interaction of two systems (either real or ideal), either of them can be understood as the model of the other system inasmuch as one represents the other [10]. As the nature of IG is a one-dimensional time-extended structure that allows for omitting the distance (measurement) concept in the mental image structure, it is our perception that further computations in this field can be done by using mathematical tools of topological spaces, which make it possible to assess the proximity of the points, while ignoring the concept of distance [11]. We believe that this approach offers good opportunities for the description, study and modeling of the "modal relationships that exist between spatial patterns, coherence laws…, regardless of the relationships between the measures and values" (Listing, 1847) [12].

Integrated behavioral units are structurally identical regular sequences, which, regardless of the IG content and the end result achieved through MG, have characteristics of bijection where each element of one set correlates with an element of another set. Due to the bijection that retains the object as an information matrix in representation of the coded structure, these structures can be understood as being isomorphic [13]. Present during BU actualization is an equivalent, time symmetrical BU derivative structure of the hemodynamic scalar gradient, with morphophysiological parameters; this structure is a continuous representation of this gradient, a biophysical equivalent of each structurally identical regular sequence (BU), a marker of the relationship that we define as translation symmetry. Therefore, it is our understanding that the integrated BU, including the biophysical equivalent, can be defined as a psychophysiological metamer in the behavioral continuum both for tactical and strategic (sums of interval-slotted interims and continuously sequenced goals) purposes.

Significant parameter fluctuations exceeding the "normal zone" boundaries—the homeostasis pattern initiating MG and characterized by a totality of its own values and vectors of all the components of the space-time configuration—include excited receptors, neural circuits, mental structures, metabolic systems and efferent mechanisms. In the MG dynamics, the parameters of homeostatic metabolism are actual numbers (representing continuous values), which in the homeostatic continuum constitute the predetermined nature of the dynamic scalar, filled-in, 4-dimensional space. Therefore, we project that it is possible to create a structural pattern corresponding to the scalar differential equation and to make a subsequent mathematical computation of the "fragments" of the psychophysiological metamer, BU having modal characteristics and existing in the dynamic scalar field. We also understand that the suggestions offered above open up new opportunities for computation of artificial intelligence models.

By defining IG and MG, we also explain the dynamics and interaction between the one-dimensional, time-extended structures generated by the fluctuating adaptive changes in homeostasis and structures in the hemodynamic biophysical equivalent, which are created by dynamic changes in the concentrations, charges, relationship mix, etc., of the physical particles and their combinations constituting the substances of metabolism. The primary interaction of the entire spectrum of these substances (with their own relationship constants) occurs under the following conditions: *sizes- 10^{-9}m (Na-0.42 μm, K-133 μm, H2O-0.276 μm, etc.); weight – 10^{-27}kg (Na - 22.99; K-39.09; H20-29.9, etc.).*

Conclusion

Having no other known size parameters, barring the time parameter IG includes all the possible and depictable types of space and measurements, which permits forming an assumption regarding their existence (possible building) in the mental formations of a human being where they occur in a compact condition and can be decoded (constructed) by the operating systems of the brain (thinking, imagination, etc.). For IG elements ("inward"), it acts as a space-time structure with an unlimited (unknown to us) number of levels of freedom.

The existence of the translation symmetry of the metabolic dynamics of homeostasis and the psychophysiological structures of the brain (IG, MG) makes it possible to extrapolate mathematical computations of the markers: the scalar (hemodynamic equivalent of MG) and the vector (subjective time) markers to the core component of the metamer of the integrated BU—the ideal IG.

Taking into account the one-dimensional nature of the ideal IG, which has an unlimited number of levels of freedom and sets the basic characteristics for the structure, vector and behavioral continuum metamer duration, we concluded that the elements of the "string theory" (M-theory) mathematical apparatus used to compute one-dimensional extended structures setting the characteristics of weight, charge, etc. (including the dual transformation providing the switchover between the different scale systems) could be used for the mathematical description of the integrated behavioral unit, motivational gradient and the ideal IG. Due to the mathematical apparatus of the basic components of the integrated BU, we will be able to identify the mathematical equivalents of the interaction mediator and relationship constant of the ideal IG, using the biophysical and time "markers". When put into practice, our suggestions (or part of them) will help to solve the problem of adequacy in the modeling of complex systems, to complement the existing research methodologies and modeling of the human psyches and artificial intelligence by using computational conclusive methods, including a mathematical analysis of the ideal mental structures.

References

1. Hayes-Roth B. An architecture for adaptive intelligent systems. Artificial Intelligence 1995; 72(l-2):329 -365.
2. Anochin PK. Philosophical aspects of the theory of the functional systems. Moscow: Science; 1978.
3. Sudakov K.V. Functional systems. Moscow: RAMS (Russian Academy of Medical Sciences) Publishing House; 2011.
4. Shvyrkov VB. Introduction to objective psychology. Neuronal basics of psychics. Moscow, Psychology Institute of RAS; 1995.
5. Kruglov AG, Gebel GY, Vasilyev AY. Impact of Intra-Extracranial Hemodynamics on Cerebral Ischemia by Arterial Hypertension (Part 1). Int J Biomed. 2012; 2(2):89-95
6. Kruglov AG et al. Psychological image as an active distributed system. Journal of International scientific Publications: Material, Methods and Technologies. 2014: 808-811.
7. Rubin AB. Kinetics of biological processes. Soros Educational Journal. 1998; 10:84-91.
8. Kruglov AG, Gebel GY, Vasilyev AY. Intracranial venous pressure as a possible determinant of mental regulation. Int J Biomed. 2011; l(4):245-8.
9. Rubinshtein SL. Fundamentals of general psychology. St. Petersburg; 2003.
10. Simankov VS, Lutsenko YeV. Adaptive management of complex systems by using the image recognition theory. Krasnodar Technological University; 1999.
11. Engelking R. General Topology. Moscow: Mir; 1986.
12. Kolmogorov AN, Yushkevich AP. Mathematics of the 19th century. Theory of analytical functions. Moscow: Science; 1981(2):98-99.
13. Vereshchagin NK, Shen A. Fundamentals of the set theory. Lectures on mathematical logic and algorithm theory Part 1. 2nd ed. Moscow: MCNMO; 2002.

CHAPTER 5.

PSYCHOPHYSIOLOGY OF A MYTHOLOGEM AS A DETERMINANT OF GOAL-DIRECTED BEHAVIOR

In accordance with modern ideas set out in the research of a number of authors, mythologem (ML) is generally regarded as a figurative, symbolic way to display reality, which is required when does not fit into a formal logic and abstract display. ML is a stable construct, generally reflecting reality in the form of sensory-specific association perceived as objective reality [1]. Man lives in the power of illusion, which is so strong that it seems as normal consciousness [2]. ML is capable of directing the activity of the individual and mobilizing this activity to achieve significant goals [3].

The objective of this study was to build a model of ML as a psychogenic stable construction having psychologycal, electrical, magnetic, hemodynamic and timing parameters of the neural networks (associations) that provide the formation, the initiation and the existence of the ML. Understanding the concept of the formation and stability of ML will help in finding the antithesis of the confidence [4] in the invincibility of ML.

Materials and methods

To create the model of ML as a meaningful unity of the neural networks having the psychologycal, electrical, magnetic, hemodynamics and timing parameters, we used our own previously published data (discussing the parameters of hemodynamics and biochemistry of the brain obtained by invasive methods) [5-8]) and data of other authors.

Discussion

ML fixates the sequence, the order of the representation elements about the reality, and serves as the conceptual basis of behavior that allows us to functionally consider ML as a “motive” for specific forms of behavior. The motive is the cause of behavior and consists of a set of dispositions, the most important of which is the need [9]. A need is defined as a state of dissatisfaction of the organism (the personality) and a deficit of what is required to maintain homeostatic balance of the organism (the personality). A special feature of "organized matter" is the selectivity of the reaction that is the subject of urgent needs, i.e. elimination of the gradient between the current status and the target status, the result for which the activity is undertaken, namely, the image of the future results generated by the subject, defined as image of the goal (IG). IG is a leading element of the conscious regulatory process. We think it possible, within ML modeling, to determine the partial identity of the ML and IG (ML~IG).

Association of the interneurons activated to provide goal-directed behavior (GDB), whose ultimate aim is the achievement of parametric equalization and the state of homeostatic balance, we consider as a possible substrate for ML as the long- term circular structure [5]. We believe that the periodic afferent stimulation, which has a constant parametric set during the exposure time (the invariant sensory pattern – training, persuasion, suggestion, etc.) is the initial step in the formation of ML(IG). The sensory afferent stimulation of synapses by the repetitive, monotonous sensory patterns (short- and long-term potentiation) creates the "beaten paths" to facilitate the passage of this particular set of patterns. The formation of the neural "beaten paths" during a quite long afferentation leads to the creation of the sustainable neuronal formation – a dominant center (DC). A DC with the properties of persistence, the concentration of an excitation from other nerve centers, the inhibition of functionally incompatible centers (i.e. filtering the input parameters of the sensory information) determines the nature of the current reactions to the time of its existence. We believe that this consistently structured neural formation creates the IG. It should be noted that the mind has the ability to create the pathological dominants, determinants, and systems [10], and to design images which do not reflect the reality but are accompanied by the sensory, cognitive and behavioral equivalents with preserved consciousness (phantom pain, some hallucinatory syndromes).

The activity of neurons reflects their involvement in the system, where the organization of all process is the informative equivalent of the result, i.e. the future [9]). The completion of the IG construction as a result of the successive sensory stimulation, in our opinion, is subjectively experienced as a state known by definition as "insight". The IG creation activates the efferent structure described by us [5] as a motivational gradient

(MG). The ultimate goal of MG implemented through GDB, is to achieve the status of parametric (homeostatic) balance. The achievement of the expected utilitarian goals (food, sexual behavior, etc) leads to the restoration of homeostasis, i.e. elimination of the MG. In contrast to the short-term and "tactical" goals, the forward-looking plans for achievement of the "strategic" goals covering large time intervals have the discrete structure of MG and the subjective time (ST) (i.e. phenomena, accompanied by the expected changes in the parameters as a result of GDB, may be formed in the interval-separated time periods, at same time being in the plot(story)-caused sequence of the events) [5].

ML, being a set of universalized symbols, has an ambivalent nature, being both a complete construct and an integral part (element) of the new constructs. Two main interacting elements of a symbol, an image and a meaning, exist only inside of the interpretations [11] where the bijective isomorphic coordinate accordance of any operational IG to the final (ideal) IG is impossible. At the same time, there is convincing evidence of a homomorphism, where full compliance with the ideal IG is impossible, but some degree of similarity is achieved. In the absence of the concretized and utilitarian form (image) during our movement to a symbolic goal, new coordinating and interpretive combinations of IG and a semantic content are formed, which create a fractional and operative image without the possibility of reaching the ideal IG. Consequently, the movement towards a symbolic goal (ML) which has not the specifics of the utilitarian goals and time constraints, creates a new degree of similarity and cannot be completed. In other words, the ML construct has the nature of the expected IG located outside of the actual achievable goal.

Considering the vector of GDB as the direction of a speedy change in the scalar variables, whose values are changed from one point in space to another, we define a "zero" (starting) point of ST in the structure of ML on the expected result of the action, i.e. IG. In psychologycal time, only the expected outcome (goal), having fixed coordinate specifications, can be taken as an abstract point (which is in the future), while the present is always a certain time interval [12]. Thus, the IG formation is a psychophysiological stimulus and starting point in the formation of the grading scale of the result achievement, namely, ST. Perhaps a prediction exists as a principle (probably genetic) of the formation of an organism (the personality). In 1930, G.E.Coghill [13] described how during embryogenesis the anatomical structures are formed long before their demand in future behavior (anticipatory structure versus the function). Several authors [14] have described the neurobiological basis of the phenomenon of the "mental anticipatory response". IG formation demonstrates the "anticipatory function" versus the structure.

MG/IG formed by the repetitive patterns of sensory impact on the object has expected time of existence until the achievement of the ultimate goal, the elimination of the imbalance and the restoration of the parametric equilibrium of the homeostasis. The fundamental properties of the living organisms belonging to the open nonequilibrium systems are their vibrational nature. The organism as a unified formation exists due to the synchronization of the rhythmic changes (the adaptive oscillation) at all hierarchical levels, from the molecular-cellular level to the organism level. Since the ultimate goal (IG) is unattainable, it is impossible to eliminate the imbalance and the restore the homeostatic balance, regardless of the amplitude and duration of the adaptive vibrational changes. The existence of the permanent IG/ML inducing the vector activity initiates the "vibrational" search for forms and vectors of GDB, which is implemented by the cognitive and behavioral activity. The strategies of the IG/ML implementation with (slightly) ineffective negative reverse relations and the conservation (increasing) of the reverse positive relations (filtration of the input sensory information), result in a loss of the correction-concordance of the GDB stages to the intrasystem and integrative mechanisms of the central nervous system. In addition, the amplitude of the adaptive and search oscillation of homeostasis decreases, a resistance increases, and the system becomes rigid. The natural result is the development of various forms and degrees of change in thinking and consciousness, as well as reduced energy potential and other manifestations of a long homeostatic imbalance and desynchronosis.

The formation of the activity of the neuronal association in the form of the electrodynamic structure (EDS) circulating through the neural network until the achievement of the result is accompanied by the metabolic support of the exchange fields of the activated neurons [8]. The electrical field of the neuron is largely flattened for the external registrars due to nonlinear dissemination of EDS and the electrical insulating properties of the membranes, astrocytes and meninges, which perhaps explains the still existing differences in EEG decoding. The increase in blood flow (i.e. number and speed of blood flows) through the vessels of the brain tissue is an hemodynamic equivalent of this activity. In the tissue in the cortex and white matter of the brain, the regional linear (in the radial vessels) and local (functional hyperemia) streams of the charged particles of blood are intensified. In accordance with V.P.Oleinik [15], the blood is regarded as an electrolyte, while the bloodstream is regarded as a conductor placed in an external magnetic field. In a moving conducting fluid, the ponderomotive forces directed perpendicular to the linear movement of the blood – the magneto-hydrodynamic forces (a magnetic dipole) - are formed. Magnetic properties of blood flow (electrolytes), having an essentially linear (radial vessels) character in the regionally supply of increased metabolism of the exchange fields of brain tissue and spreading perpendicularly to the axial potential do not have the insulating barriers in the form of biological tissue, as an interaction with intracerebral structures, as well as for external recorders. In biological systems, the effect of an induction occurs under impact of the extremely weak (nano- and picotesla) alternating magnetic fields, where primary receptor is a water-salt component, while the primary target is the nuclear spin of hydrogen atoms [16].

The alternating electric fields, with the parameters imitating the Schumann's resonances (Konig, 1974: cited by Lednev VV et al. [16]) and defining the circadian rhythms (Wever, 1974: cited by Lednev VV et al. [16]), influence the psychophysical condition of the person. The match between the Schumann resonance frequency and the alpha-rhythm of the human brain (7.83 Hz) suggested that the response to the external action depends on a matching (resonance) with frequency parameters which are identical (close) to the characteristics of the intracerebral electrical and magnetic dipoles (the neural circuits, including an inactive).

The data of Konig, Wever et al. (1974), in our opinion, reflect the external manifestation of the activity of neuronal structures of the first signal system of the brain activated due to external influences: an induction by external magnetic fields. We believe that the main mechanism of this interaction is a response of the brain (neurons) structures with electromagnetic properties (dipoles) to the external stimulus with identical (close) frequency characteristics (resonance). In the absence of the primary afferent sensory information from the known receptors, we consider the possibility of the direct resonance effect on the neural structures of the brain during exposure to the external magnetic field with the actualization of the brain dipoles coinciding in the frequency characteristics. A demonstrative example of this effect, possibly related to the unconditioned reflexes, in our opinion, is animals sensing that an earthquake is about to happen and fleeing from it, even at a distance of 200 km from the epicenter. Thus, by our assumption, the initiator of mental activity, along with the sensor variables, may be an external vector of magnetic induction with the effect of a direct impact (resonance) on the neuronal circuits (magnetic dipoles) of the brain.

We believe that the registration of the magnetic fields arising during the activation of mental activity largely relates to the parameters of the resulting multipole magnetic field that is a result of vector addition of magnetic dipoles: EDS of the activated neural associations and regional vessels (interdependent distributed systems) having different latency intervals and angular vector differences. We also believe that the differences in the genesis of the magnetic induction should be considered during detailed coding of the result of the magnetographic mapping.

ML, in our opinion, may have objective, measurable parameters: 1) voltage variation of the magnetic fields of the brain of different origin; 2) hemodynamic equivalent with a change in blood flow and shape of the vessels in the exchange fields of the activated neurons in the veins and venules of the brain tissue with a diameter of 60 – 250 microns [5].

In this work, deliberately simplifying the structure of the components, we considered only the most general principles of the structural construction of ML and the gradient behavior under the influence of ML. Our follow-up works will be focused on the following issues: effects of the methods of external influence, which create and initiate ML formation; the filtration of the input information; the transformation of the character traits of the individual under the ML impact; the priority of ML mainstreaming; tunnelization of thinking and narrowing of consciousness; ML interaction and influence on unconditioned reflex behavior; and objectification of ML markers.

Conclusion

Regarding MLs as complexes of psychologycal, electrical, magnetic, hemodynamic, and temporary equivalents, we define them as properties of a unified psychogenic construct initiating GDB to achieve the ultimate goal: the homeostatic balance of the subject. Localization of the starting point of ST, the timescale for the rate of the result achievement on ML/IG that is located outside accessibility, determines the coordinates of the actualization of the structures of GDB, which are unable to achieve the ultimate goal.

We believe that anticipatory, prospective formation of IG, initiating adaptive forms of behavior, is a manifestation of a general principle of "anticipatory response" (the formation of the future in the present moment) inherent for somatic and mental spheres of human ontogenesis.

References

1. Jung KG. *Archetype and Symbol.* M.: Canon; 1991.
2. Berdyaev NA. *Slavery and Freedom*. M.: ACT; 2006.
3. Toporkov AL. *Myth: tradition and psychology of perception. The myth and mythology in modern Russia*. Moscow; 2000.
4. Cassirer E. Technique of modern political myths. Vestn Moscow State University. 1990; (Ser. 7, Philosophy) 2:58-65.
5. Kruglov AG, Gebel GY, Vasilyev AY. Intracranial venous pressure as a possible determinant of mental regulation. Int J Biomed. 2011; 1(4):245-8.
6. Kruglov AG, Gebel GY, Vasilyev AY. Impact of intra-extracranial hemodynamics on cerebral ischemia by arterial hypertension (Part 1 and Part 2) Int J Biomed. 2012; 2(2):89-101.
7. Kruglov A, Vasilyev AYu. Mathematical approaches in studying the ideal image of the goal. Int J Biomed. 2014; 4(1):46-48.
8. Kruglov A, Vasilyev AYu. Psychological image as an active distributed system. J Int Scien Publ Mat Met Tech. 2014; 8:808-11.
9. Shvyrkov VB. *Introduction to objective psychology. Neuronal basics of psychics.* Moscow: Psychology Institute of RAS; 1995.
10. Kryzhanovsky GN. *Discirculatory pathology of the nervous system.* M.: Medinformagenstvo; 2009.
11. Losev AF. *Essays on ancient symbolism and mythology*. M.:Nauka; 1993.
12. Rubinshtein SL. *Fundamentals of general psychology*. St. Petersburg; 2003.
13. Coghill GE. Correlated anatomical and physiological studies of the growth of the nervous system of amphibia. The mechanism of association of *Amblystoma punctatum*. J Comp Neurol. 1930; 51:311-375.
14. Rajewski KS, Georgiev VP. Mediator amino acids: neurochemical and neuropharmacological aspects. Moscow; 1986.
15. Oleinik VP. *Fundamentals of the interaction of physical fields with biological substances.* Kharkiv: National Aerospace University; 2006.
16. Lednev VV, Belova NA, Rozhdestvenskaya ZE, Tyros KhP. Biological effects of weak variable magnetic fields and biological precursors of earthquakes. Geophysical Processes and the Biosphere. 2003; 2(1):3-11.

Alexander Kruglov, Alexander Vasilyev, Veronica Sherman

Human Dynamic Homeostasis Control Matrix in the Norm with Psychophysiological Aspects

Published by International Medical Research and Development Corporation

ISBN: 978-0-692-61998-8

10 9 8 7 6 5 4 3 2 1

Printed in the United States of America
2016

Made in United States
North Haven, CT
05 November 2026

21796509R00036